Intermittent Fasting:

How to Eat what you want and still have rapid weight loss and gain lean muscle for beginners

By

Heather Trill

professional before attempting any techniques outlined in this book.

By reading this document, the reader agrees that under no circumstances are is the author responsible for any losses, direct or indirect, which are incurred as a result of the use of information contained within this document, including, but not limited to, —errors, omissions, or inaccuracies.

Table of Contents

Introduction

Unless you're one of the lucky few people on the planet who can eat whatever they want but never seem to gain an ounce, you've likely been on a diet or two.

And with so many fad diets to choose from - the grapefruit diet, the cabbage soup diet, the raw food diet and the juice diet, each more bland and painful than the one that came before it – you probably found one that helped you lose a pound or two.

But based on the history of most diets, those pesky extra pounds are likely to be still hanging around, as stubborn as ants at a summer picnic.

That's because most fad dieters find that whilst their latest diet will temporarily help them to drop a few pounds, it doesn't teach them lasting changes, so in almost all cases, the weight just comes creeping back on again, usually with a vengeful few extra pounds, just to teach us a little lesson.

So, it's back to the books and back to the diets, only to lose – and gain – all over again.

What this book covers:

We will look at some of the benefits that we gain to fasting in addition to what Intermittent Fasting is all about. We will also look at what Intermittent Fasting is all about and what exactly it entails.

If there's one thing experts agree on, that the cycle of yo-yo dieting wreaks havoc on the metabolism, slowing it down to a crawl and making losing weight that much more difficult in the future.

So, is it all over but the crying, and should you just head to the kitchen and whip up a batch of double-fudge brownies and forget about it?

Well, no, don't throw the towel in just yet. There are things you can do to stop the viscous cycle and rev up your metabolic rate again.

With intermittent fasting, you can drop weight quickly, without feeling too deprived along the way.

"For body transformation, intermittent fasting works." This book contains some of the useful tips on how to achieve a successful fast and in the right manner, read on to be enlightened more.

Chapter 1: All about Intermittent Fasting

Intermittent fasting is not a starvation diet. On the other hand, it's also not a way to eat a steady diet of junk food and get away with it. Intermittent fasting is a planned schedule of eating that allows you to eat a normal, healthy diet most of the time, and then requires you to spend a short period of time-consuming far less food. There are some intermittent fasting plans that divide fasting and non-fasting periods into mere hours, such as eight hours of eating followed by twelve or sixteen hours of fasting.

More commonly, intermittent fasts are divided by days of the week.

On the Intermittent Fast Diet, you eat a "normal" diet for five days of the week, interspersed with two days of fasting. Although the research on intermittent fasting is still in

the beginning stages, there is sufficient evidence that eating in this way can help to shed fat, regulate some of the hormones associated with obesity and hunger, and even improve overall cholesterol levels.

Because intermittent fasting can have a beneficial effect on the hormones that stimulate fat storage and hunger, it can be a very useful strategy for losing weight and shedding body fat. It can also be a very good way for people who don't otherwise follow a healthy diet to break addictions to foods that are unhealthy and learn to make healthier food choices overall.

On the Intermittent Fast Diet, you eat a healthy diet that is close or equal to your daily caloric requirements for five out of seven days. On the two fasting days, women consume 500 calories per day while men consume 600 calories. Because you'll still be eating during the fasting days, this method of intermittent fasting does not generally lead to overeating on non-fasting days, which can be an unwelcome side effect of other fasting plans.

Fasting isn't something new. Human beings have been fasting for a large part of history due to food scarcity or religious/spiritual reasons. Nowadays people fast a lot less than before, and this is quite logical with all the food we have access to.

Intermittent Fasting, on the other hand, is quite new. It is a new and different way of planning your meals. Research has shown several benefits regarding our health and

longevity when you Intermittent Fast. It has shown that it, when done properly, manages our body weight, extends life, regulates blood glucose and a lot more. Normally we are accustomed to eating three meals a day, and maybe even consume snacks in-between those meals. But Intermittent Fasting is different. With Intermittent Fasting you are consciously choosing to skip certain meals. This can be done one day a week, but it can also mean that you skip breakfast every day and that lunch will be your first meal of the day. There are several ways to do it, but this really depends on your goals.

The meaning of Intermittent Fasting is that you deprive yourself of food on certain points of the day. You will only eat between certain hours, the so-called 'Time Windows'. You will choose these time windows by what suits you best throughout your day. For example, if you choose to eat from 12:00 PM to 08:00 PM, then that will be your time window. You'll make sure that you consume all your calories in those hours and nothing outside of them.

How many meals you eat is also up to you. You can choose to divide all your food between 5 or 6 meals, but you can also choose to eat 1 or 2 meals. Regardless, the main concept is: consuming all your calories between certain hours (your time window). So, Intermittent Fasting is not a diet, it is just a different way of consuming your calories. It has nothing to do with what you eat, but is about when you eat. Of course, you need to eat healthy foods and make sure that you don't overeat in the first place in order to be healthy, but Intermittent Fasting itself provides for great benefits.

Chapter 2: Who to and not to fast

Who Should and Should Not Try Intermitt ent Fasting?

Most people can safely follow the Intermittent Fast Diet; however, you should consult your doctor before beginning the diet, since it is not recommended for some people.

People Who Are Not Good Candidates for the Intermittent Fast Diet

In particular, women who are pregnant or nursing should not attempt intermittent fasting. The calorie guidelines for the fasting days are simply too low. However, once you have had your baby and/or have finished nursing, intermittent fasting can help you get your pre-pregnancy body back.

People with type 2 diabetes should not undertake this diet. Although some evidence shows that it may correct imbalances of or insensitivity to insulin, once type 2 diabetes has been diagnosed, fasting is not advised.

People with a history of eating disorders should not go on a fasting diet. If you feel that you may have an eating disorder or that you're at risk of developing one, it is not recommended that you try the Intermittent Fast Diet.

Children and adolescents should not go on the Intermittent Fast Diet. Please consult a pediatrician or nutritionist if you are seeking a weight-loss plan for anyone under eighteen years of age.

People Who Are Well-Suited for the Intermittent Fast Diet

The Intermittent Fast Diet can be a great plan for anyone who is otherwise healthy but would like to lose weight and shed body fat. However, the format of the diet can make it especially beneficial to some specific groups of people.

People whocurrently eat an unhealthy diet:

People who eat a good deal of fast food, processed foods, and sugar can benefit from the Intermittent Fast Diet's nutritionally balanced approach. The focus of both fasting and non- fasting days is on whole foods: primarily lean meats, fresh fruits and vegetables, low-fat dairy, and whole grains. Many people find that after eating this type of diet for a few weeks, they are better able to appreciate healthier whole foods and have a better understanding of what makes a well-rounded diet.

People who are addicted to sugary foods or empty calories:

Many people become addicted to sugary foods, high-carbohydrate processed snacks, and empty calorie beverages such as sodas and blended coffee drinks, which have lots of calories and little to no nutrition. For some of these people, the Intermittent Fast Diet can have the added benefit of helping them break those addictions. This is not only because of the focus on whole foods but also because of the calorie restrictions on fasting days. When you only have 500 to 600 calories to use in a day, it's hard to justify spending half of it on one cola. After a week or two of living without those foods, many people report that the cravings and withdrawal symptoms sub- side.

People who need an especially simple plan:

Some people just naturally do better when steps and choices are very limited. A diet with too many variations and choices or that requires too much planning and decision- making are often hard for such people to maintain. The Intermittent Fast Diet is simple, straightforward, and mapped out step by step. Because of calorie limitations, the fasting day meal plans are extremely simple, and recipes often have just a few ingredients.

Chapter 3: Myths behind Intermittent Fasting

With all the information regarding fitness and nutrition floating on the web, it can be very easy to lose sight of what is real and what is fiction. The recommendations regarding which diet you should implement varies a lot; many are valid, but there are also some common myths.

Not knowing that those myths are false, people can implement the wrong advice, thus sabotaging their own progress (while having a very good work ethic). Me personally, I get very upset when I see this. I used to be the newbie who would search every forum of the web, getting very excited about implementing the false advice that I would receive. And in the end I would sabotage my own progress.

Eventually I slowly began to see that many myths regarding nutrient and Intermittent Fasting just weren't true. But it was when I found mentors who had the results that I wanted that I fully understood what I needed to do to get the same results as them. To be honest though, to get to the point where I could fully see which advice was false and which wasn't was very time-consuming and frustrating. I want to spare you this process by debunking the common Intermittent

Fasting myths. But before I dive into it, let me explain why and how myths are formed:

1. Lack of Knowledge and/or Interest.

With all newly discovered scientific evidence, there are people who want to draw conclusions on it while lacking the knowledge needed to properly do so. In order for them to properly draw conclusions on the results of a particular study, they first need an academic background in that specific field. Most of the time they don't have one, so they simply draw conclusions that are false. Besides that, there are people who have the proper knowledge, but who just repeat the same thing over and over again (while somewhat knowing that it is incorrect).

This usually happens when people lose interest in the specific field they are studying and don't want to put in the effort to properly draw conclusions on a particular result. Another main reason is that scientists are afraid of losing credibility. It is very embarrassing for scientists to admit that they were wrong about a certain subject when they discover that the opposite of what they are preaching is true. Most of the time scientists won't publish their newly discovered results in order to retain their credibility.

2. Social Conditioning

When you repeat a lie enough, it eventually becomes the truth. If you keep hearing something that isn't (or is) true, you will eventually think that it must be true. This is also called social conditioning. Why is that? Because we as human beings don't have enough energy or time to actually test everything out ourselves. We need others to 'invent the wheel' for us, so that we can focus on other, more important things. So, while social conditioning can be very helpful, it can also sabotage us. At some point, when these socially conditioned myths are spread enough, it will be very hard to go against it and discover the truth.

3. (False) Marketing

Supplement, food and fitness companies are constantly trying to sell us products by presenting false information. These companies benefit greatly from people who don't have enough knowledge about fitness or nutrition, because they are easier to manipulate. They use manipulation and lies to falsely promote their products to people who aren't well informed. For example, the grain industry is constantly claiming that you need to begin your day with a healthy (read: filled with sugar) cereal, or the food industry which is constantly saying that you need to feed your body throughout the day benefit from the people who think that they constantly need to buy large quantities of food.

The common myths about Intermittent Fasting are the following:

Myth 1: You Will Be Hungry While Fasting

Most people who hear about Intermittent Fasting for the first time are afraid of being hungry while fasting. While this might be true for the beginning when you try to implement Intermittent Fasting, this will undoubtedly go away very quickly. Why is that? Well, almost everything that we do in our day-to-day lives are formed habits. We have habits so that the body doesn't need to use willpower to do certain things. Having said that, when your body is giving you a signal that you are hungry, it is actually a habit trigger.

Most of the time you aren't really hungry, but because you normally eat at that moment you will receive a habit trigger. When you first implement Intermittent Fasting, it will be difficult to ignore these hunger triggers. This is because it takes around 30-60 days to form a new habit or remove an old one. If you persist for the first 60 days, it will become much easier to ignore these signals and they will even eventually go away. Your body will then send hunger signals to different parts of the day. So, when you start implementing Intermittent Fasting, be sure to ignore the hunger signals you receive outside of your time windows for at least the first 60 days. When you do this effectively, your body will learn to send hunger signals to different parts of the day.

Myth 2: Intermittent Fasting Causes Nutrient Deficiencies

Many people think that you won't receive enough vitamins when you are fasting, but this is not true. When you are fasting, you are 'teaching' your body to eat at certain intervals. By doing this, you will not lose essential vitamins and/or minerals. Besides, the nutrients you lose in a day of fasting are regained again when you eat.

Also, you can take your dose of vitamins by taking pills containing them if you really want to consume our vitamins at certain times of the day.

Myth 3: You Are Starving Yourself On Purpose

Nowadays, we are quick to label 'missing certain meals' as starving yourself. We are so accustomed to having food around us 24/7 that we freak out when we skip a meal. Yet I wouldn't call 'skipping a meal' the same as 'starving yourself'. True starvation is when your body depletes all its fat stores and begins to consume your muscles for energy, which leads to death very quickly.

With Intermittent Fasting though, this is not the case. The fasting periods are very short and you get enough calories from your meals (besides your fat stores) to sustain your energy levels.

Myth 4: Intermittent Fasting Will Have A Negative Effect On Your Weight Training Performance

Another myth brought into the world without real and legitimate evidence to back it up. Research done by several people who were fasting during Ramadan concludes that aerobic activities had an insignificant negative effect on their performance. This is even while being dehydrated, as Ramadan involves restriction of fluids.

More studies that didn't involve the restriction of fluids have found that strength training is unaffected by fasting, even when the individual is fasting for 3 days straight. So, that people think that they can't perform well while in a fasted state is simply not true.

Myth 5: You Need To Eat Small Meals throughout the Day to Keep Your Blood Sugar Levels under Control

Some 'health experts' claim that eating small meals will help you to control your blood sugar. But the thing is, blood sugar levels are well-regulated and maintained when you are healthy. They don't go up and down that much when you go without food for a couple of hours, or even a day.

Also, if you look at it from an evolutionary perspective, it is totally normal to go without food for a couple of hours, days, or even a week. Our ancestors sometimes had to go through times where they didn't have any food available, and this didn't have a big impact on their blood sugar levels. So, the myth that you need to eat small meals throughout the day to keep your blood sugar levels under control is simply not true.

Myth 6: You Will Mostly Lose Muscle and Little Fat When You Fast

The exact opposite is true. Fat is a high energy molecule and it contains far more energy than protein (it is around 2 times more energy dense than protein). Therefore, it makes sense for the body to first use the stored fats as an energy source than protein. Also, the primary purpose of fat is to be an energy reservoir for us when food is scarce.

The proteins in our muscles contain a lot less energy, so it isn't efficient for the body to use protein as an energy source. Also, the main purpose of protein is more critical for our skeletal muscle and for our bodies to function properly instead of providing the body with energy. Additionally, if you compare the calorie reserves that are in fats and proteins, you see a tremendous difference. About 85% of our calorie reserves are in fat stores and 14% of protein. Obviously, fat is the most important energy storage molecule. So, from a physiological standpoint, it makes sense for our bodies to first go to our fat stores for energy when food is scarce.

Myth 7: It Is Bad For You When You Skip Breakfast, And It Also Will Make You Fat

It is true that people who skip breakfast are more likely to be fat. This is due the fact that most breakfast skippers have inconsistent eating habits and show a lot less concern for their health. Another reason why people who skip breakfast are heavier than those who don't, is that people who skip breakfast are more likely to be on a diet. And being on a diet can lead to binge eating. Also, people who diet tend to be heavier than non-dieters in the first place.

Therefore, it is logical that most people think that skipping breakfast itself makes you fat. But as explained earlier, it is what breakfast skippers do besides skipping breakfast that makes them fat, and not the actual skipping of the breakfast itself.

Myth 8: Fasting is bad for women

Some people like to argue that Intermittent Fasting is bad for women. People think that it can negatively affect hormone levels and glucose tolerance as well as lead to decreased satisfaction and frequent hunger in women. While some studies support that theory, other studies have shown that women may continue practicing Intermittent Fasting without any effect on their bodies or hunger levels.

As a woman, I can attest that sometimes, I am just sick of dieting, but that has something to do more with when I was counting macronutrients and my calorie intake than my practicing Intermittent Fasting. I love Intermittent Fasting. I have more control of how much I take into my body and feel like I am able to achieve more satisfaction with my meals if I can intake more due to my fasting throughout the day.

Do I miss eating breakfast? Not really. I miss eating breakfast foods at fast food restaurants, which are bad for you anyway. I can still eat breakfast foods for dinner or lunch if I want. Sure, I cannot get that chorizo biscuit from Carl's Jr that may be bad for my body and daily calorie intake, but I can always make something like it at home for cheaper with fewer calories. I prefer skipping breakfast anyway so that I can train fasted and not worry about packing or making breakfast before work. Who needs extra work in the morning? That is just time taken away from me playing with my phone or sleeping in!

Myth 9: Fasted Training is bad for you

There was a time when people thought fasted training was great for burning fat, especially if you -are performing cardio. Professional weightlifters were worried that fasted training can cause catabolism, which is the breaking down of muscle. This is also the reason why some athletes attempt to consume something about 30 minutes after a workout so that they can meet a "metabolic window."

Recent studies have showed that even 60 minutes of running while fasted will insignificantly affect your muscle growth. Fasted training will not negatively affect your strength performance as once was thought. However, there is still some unease when it comes to fasted weight training due to the ability to synthesize protein. To help aid in the synthesizing of proteins, it is recommended to consume up to 10mg of BCAA (branched chain amino acids) before and after weight training.

Myth 10: Eating Large Meals at Night Will Make You Gain Weight

You may have heard this saying before: "Eat like a king in the morning, eat like a prince for lunch, and eat like a pauper for dinner." What does that even mean? It basically means eat your smallest meals at night and your biggest meals in the morning. The idea is that consuming large meals at night make you gain a lot of weight. While, eating large amounts of carbs at night will make you weigh more in the morning than if you were to consume just protein; that is only due to the fact that consuming more carbs means your body will retain more water.

More carbs mean more water weight. That makes sense, doesn't it? Carbohydrates tend to hold onto more water than proteins or fats. Recent studies have shown that consuming large meals at night does not make you gain more fat. Actually, recent studies have shown that your meal times do not matter. Have you not eaten throughout the day? Then feel free to eat at night. If you feel like just fasting throughout the day and eating one meal at night, feel free to. The professional competitive eater, Sonya Thomas, also known as The Black Widow, consumes one large meal at the end of a day instead of small meals throughout the day. You may think that competitive eaters are heavy set individuals, but she will definitely surprise you.

Chapter 4: Benefits of Intermittent Fasting

As they were some benefits of the fasting, there are people who are utilizing this to lose excess weight plus some are using it to raise their health problems. Some individuals also say that fasting is a strategy to look young and possess a longer life. This is why that this procedure sounds intriguing to my opinion. The simple fact is that same reasons why I would like to reveal the intermittent fasting benefits together with you.

Really, this ingesting style isn't that challenging. Accusation in court is essentially eating whatever you need within a day and then the overnight you are likely to fast. It indicates no food! (Besides water).It is very completely different from our usual eating habits. However, you can see it as being an extreme weight-loss but fasting is really a great means for anyone to search and feel great inside and outside!

Periodic fasting can help clear up the mind and strengthen the body and the spirit. Although people commonly believe that depriving yourself of food for too long is unhealthy for you, scientists have proven that Intermittent Fasting provides many benefits.

1: It Removes Food/ Sugar Cravings

A lot of the time when we feel "hungry" we actual feel cravings for sugars and carbohydrates. When you are fasting, your body will switch from using carbohydrates as fuel to using your burned fat stores instead. Your body will learn that carbohydrates aren't needed for energy and that it can use the fat already stored in your body for energy.

Aside from removing your sugar cravings, you will also remove the cravings for the food itself. Because your body "will realize" that it doesn't need food for energy, it won't crave it too often. Thus, by removing all the hunger triggers you'll get through the day. This is why the myth of "eating 5-6 times a day" is not true. When you eat 5-6 times a day and even implement carbohydrates, you'll never allow your body to burn fat. This is due the fact that the body will use the carbohydrates as energy first before using the fat in your body.

2: It Raises Insulin Sensitivity

Insulin is a hormone in the body that regulates the function of cells. Insulin is made by the pancreas and is secreted when we eat food. It then binds to signal cells and allows our body to store the sugars as energy. The less insulin we need to store these sugars, the more sensitive we become to insulin, and the better insulin can do its work in the long term.

When we eat 5 to 6 times a day, our insulin levels stay too high for a long period of time. This insulin won't be used effectively, and this will eventually raise our resistance to it. When we are resistant to insulin, we can develop type 2 diabetes or prediabetes. Diabetes is a disease that prevents us from storing all the sugars we consume, because the insulin that our pancreas produces won't work properly. When this happens the sugars will not be stored as energy and will remain in our bloodstream, leading to high blood sugar levels and hardening of the blood vessels.

This can eventually cause kidney diseases, heart attacks, erectile dysfunction, and loss of vision, strokes, nerve damage and much more critical health problems. However, when you fast for a long period of time, you are forcing your body to use the fat stored as energy and not the food that you are digesting. This will allow your body to create less insulin and therefore become more insulin sensitive, preventing all these problems.

3: It Is Very Simple Intermittent Fasting is very simple.

It doesn't require much effort to plan the quantity, quality and timing of your meals. Any active gym practitioners put much effort in preparing their meals to track their calories. This method is fine by itself, but can be very energy draining and time consuming.

In this day and age, we don't have much time anymore due to our fast-paced, demanding lifestyles, so it is better to save time by eliminating unnecessary duties like meal prepping. When you are fasting you only need to worry about 1 or 2 meals, and you always know at which times of the day you are going to eat. This will allow you to spend a greater amount of time on more important tasks.

When you realize that meal prepping is not so important, you will notice that you are still getting the same results with less effort. This is also called the 80/20 principle. 80% of our results come from 20% of our efforts. It is up to us to find out which 20% matters. And often, meal prepping doesn't belong to the 20%.

Also, because you are eating one or two large meals a say, it won't be necessary to constantly keep track of your calories. And it is much more difficult to over consume your daily calories in one or two meals (unless you are eating junk food of course).

Note: If you are a professional bodybuilder, then this doesn't apply to you. You can't expect to enter competitions and win them while not staying as lean as possible. So, for those people who are entering competitions, I highly recommend that you keep track of all your calories and stick to what works!

4: It is Flexible

Having strict meal plans can be very difficult to sustain. Most of us have important and demanding jobs that don't allow us to eat when we need to. Rather, we get breaks at the moments that we don't really need them. Or we are traveling a lot, which keeps us from eating our meals when we need to. Fasting, however, provides a huge amount of flexibility. Because you have a short time window, you can choose when to eat. This will give you the opportunity to eat when it suits you best.

For me personally, it becomes really hard to plan my meals and stay on track of my meal schedule when I am traveling or working. Fasting allows me to go without eating for a long time and simply eat when it suits me best.

5: Health Benefits

Studies show that Intermittent Fasting has many health benefits. Individuals who are overweight or suffer from diseases like diabetes may benefit the most from Intermittent Fasting.

Overweight people or individuals with type 2 diabetes will lose more weight and improve their heart health when they fast occasionally. Even if they don't reduce calorie in- take (but rather stay in maintenance mode), they will see results. But of course, if you want to maximize your results, make sure you're in a small calorie deficit and eat healthy foods.

Other health benefits are:

• Limiting inflammation

• Reducing blood pressure

• Improve pancreatic function

• Protects against cardiovascular disease

• Reduce total cholesterol and LDL levels

• Improves insulin sensitivity

While Intermittent Fasting itself is healthy for diabetic people, it can be harmful due to the fact that you are depriving yourself of nutrients at certain times of the day. So again, Intermittent Fasting is healthy for you if you are diabetic, but be sure to consult your doctor first!

6: Rapid Weight Loss

As stated earlier, normally you'll receive energy from the carbohydrates that you consume. This will prevent you from burning the fat you have stored in your body. Yet when you are fasting, you are forcing your body to use the fat you have stored for energy. This by itself will lead to instant and rapid fat loss, which means that you will not only look better, but actually be healthier too.

Also, because you are fasting for 1 or 2 days every week, you are automatically cutting many calories (1000-4500 calories a week). This will result in massive and rapid weight loss, allowing you to lose approximately 0.5-1 pound a week! You will be able to keep your muscle and lose the fat, resulting in amazing body transformations.

7: Improves Brain Health

Intermittent Fasting also has many benefits for the brain. It improves your memory functioning and accelerates learning. It also boosts your BDNF (Brain Derived Neurotropic Factor), which in turn builds your brain tissues. This will make you smarter and help you gain stronger muscles.

Some other benefits are:

Prevents Depression

Researchers have shown that having low BDNF is linked to depression. Good against Alzheimer's

Disease Research was conducted with 2 mice with Alzheimer's disease. One was Intermittent Fasting and the other mouse followed the standard diet (both were consuming the same amount of calories).

They were put in a Morris water maze, and the mouse who was Intermittent Fasting found his way much faster than the other.

Increases Ketone Production

Intermittent Fasting actively stimulates the production of ketones. Ketones are acids that are made by the body to help it use fat as an energy source instead of using carbohydrates as an energy source.

Effective against Brain Trauma

Fasting reduces the mitochondrial dysfunction, oxidative stress and cognitive decline that usually result from brain traumas.

Prevents Huntington's Disease

This disease will deplete your BDNF levels, but research showed that fasting rats with Huntington's disease kept their BDNF levels stable.

Detoxification

It is intended to cleanse the human system of toxins that accumulated during rapid fast-food and heavy meals.

Chapter 5: Does Intermittent Fasting really work?

Intermittent fasting is intended on allowing your body to be hungry enough to consume from stored energy without being in starvation. Starvation mode is when your body has lacked calories for so long that when you do eat instead of using the energy the body will immediately store it in reserves just in case another starvation happens. This is why the fad of "yo-yo dieting" was so unsuccessful – people put themselves into starvation and would actually gain weight once they began eating again. This is also why it is important to have a proper fasting schedule since you want to avoid starvation mode.

Research into weight loss has been around since the 1920's. Studies involving fasting have shown the same results with everything from fruit flies to monkeys. Fasting actually affects what you lose. Most diets will cause you to lose fat, water and even a little muscle but intermittent fasting has been shown to actually concentrate your weight loss on fat alone. It does this by choosing where the best energy source is during your fasted state. Normally your body would choose glucose in the bloodstream or temporarily stored glycogen in the liver since they are easier to process.

When you fast these become unavailable which forces the body to choose the only other stored energy available – fat. This is especially true with working out. If you have tried to drink protein shakes before a workout and have not noticed any improvement this is because your body is choosing to consume the shake rather than any excess body fat you have. Working out in a fasted state forces the body to consume fat to keep up your energy levels.

When you fast, in addition to making your body burn fat you also increase your sensitivity to insulin. When we think of insulin most people think of it as something diabetics need, the reason they need it is because either their body has become desensitized to their own or they are not producing enough. Insulin regulates the amount of glucose in the blood and those who are overweight often find their levels are not right because the body produces so much that it becomes desensitized. By fasting we can increase the sensitivity since your body is being deprived of the readily available glucose it would have from eating too often.

This is a very important tool since with desensitization your body may choose to store more of the glycogen it's making rather than burning it causing your blood glucose level to fluctuate in ways it shouldn't. As the problem of obesity grows worldwide the amount of research into dietary phenomenon grows also. Fasting has its own plethora of science behind why it really does work. So what happens on a day where you don't fast?

The regular intake of food allows the body to keep using the glucose in the bloodstream as it is energy source. Insulin sensitivity will be at normal (or in some cases desensitized) levels. Easily processable glycogen stores will be full which means any additional energy the body receives will go into storage as fat. It won't matter if you eat 20 calories or 200 over your needed amount, anything excess becomes fat and your body has no need to consume any stored energy.

Fasting can be seen as a training method, you are training your body to be more efficient in how it consumes the nutrition you give it. The physiological reasons alone are good enough, but what about the benefits that also come from losing weight? Those who weigh less enjoy a much lower risk for a variety of different health issues, they're also seen as socially superior (something controversial but unfortunately true) and the emotional benefits of having lost excess weight can also lead to an overall happier life. Weight loss can also lead to improvement in other areas – heavier people find they have bad knees or back issues from the strain of carrying extra weight.

The advantages of fasting which might be stated earlier are just the typical ones. The fact in this is a part of the benefits that are mentioned above is always that each individual who have advantages from fasting a result of the belief that everyone is exclusive. And absolutely, each individual who will about to fast will get the matter that he/she desires to be!

Intermittent fasting has grown to be quite the sensation right now. You can find were recent reports that showed that with somebody that has tried it, they dropped a few pounds, and increased how much their own health. Simply to present you with a perception, intermittent fasting is a style of eating where you stand likely to alternative your intervals of fasting, oftentimes only having water as well as on the opposite hand, non-fasting is simply eating precisely what you choose no matter how fatty food is.

Quite simply, a person can eat all sorts of things he wants throughout a 24-hour period and fast for the following 24 hours. This technique to weight control is based on the research along with the ethical practices across the world. When the person will going to present an intermittent fasting he then will certainly get what he could be wanting.

You are likely to notice that there are numerous kinds of intermittent fasts. You can find that we now have 2 kinds of intermittent fasting these are the commonly used as well as the easiest. First could be the daily fasting in which the person only grows to take in once just about every 20-28 hours within a 4-hour period.

The second reason is fasting for 1-3x every week, also referred to as different day fasting, when a man or woman eats anything he desires on a single day along with fast the entire of the following day.

Intermittent fasting has many beneficial effects as tried on wildlife like animals and also primates. A report finds out that a man who does the fasting will about to decrease the levels of insulin that he's having and will about to improve the resistance of the neurons inside the brain. In 2008, a survey was developed about intermittent fasting plus it established that the lifespan of an individual improves of 40.4% and 56.6% in C. The public that does the various day fasting has indicated that they tend to give up more weight as opposed to ones who are getting the normal diet. Along with the 2009 study showed that intermittent fasting around the rats improved the rats' survival after having a continual heart failure via pro-angiogenic and then these people have a lengthy lifespan also.

The study only caution is usually that there are few studies which have been completed to the people who do intermittent fasts. The results with the upper frequency within the composition of the body and workouts are interesting and not yet explored in your community of research. However, there are many positive results. Very last month, a study that had been made by the National Academy of Sciences posted a book that ensures that reducing calories 30% per day will planning to increase the memory perform from the old people. In the past year 2007, the journal Free Radical Biology & Medicine indicates to the public the fact that those who are having to deal with bronchial asthma who quicker had much fewer symptoms and in addition they reduction in the markers in the blood that they're having in comparison to the first.

Chapter 6: Nutrition and Training

A major part of Intermittent Fasting is eating. Yes, that sounds self-explanatory, doesn't it? Let me explain. Eating is very important in our day-to-day lives and we must consider what we consume very carefully. With Intermittent Fasting, you can consume higher calorie foods like that six-dollar burger from Carl's Jr or that pasta from Olive Garden without worrying too much about excessive fat gain, but you do have to ensure that your body gets its proper nutrients.

Even though you are using Intermittent Fasting for some flexible dieting, lower calorie foods with a high nutrition profile will help you feel full longer. It is that fiber that fills your stomach! And well, fiber also gets your system moving, if you know what I mean. If you are practicing the Alternate Day Diet or the 5:2 diet, you will find that if you consume a burger for your 500 calories, you will starve before you sleep. Yeah, that burger may taste great, but it will not fill your stomach enough. Plus, you will not get to eat the fries!

How can you get a burger without fries? On the days when you need to consume about 500 calories, it is best to consume 500 calories in vegetables because you will fill your stomach up and feel satisfied. I do not know about you, but most of the time, if I eat a small meal before bed, I will not be able to sleep. I need to eat to sleep! It sounds funny but it is true! As I mentioned in the previous section, you can still lose weight when you consume "bad" foods, but what is important is that you eat fewer calories than your body burns in a day. Do not let food consume your thoughts. If you want to eat out, go for it, but also make note that you should make healthy choices or eat healthy foods the rest of the day.

Eating junk food all day may sound appealing but the sugar and salt will definitely have you buzzing more than if you had been drinking. Speaking of drinking, try to avoid drinking your calories. Those go by fast and you will miss them when they are! Sure, you can have a Starbucks Frappuccino, but have you seen how many calories are in one? Or how much sugar is in it? My favorite drink, the caramel ribbon crunch Frappuccino, in a Venti size without whipped cream can be over 60 grams of sugar. Seriously, beware!

Also, it is really important to remember that while alcohol can be great, it can have some negative side effects. Alcohol is an empty calorie drink which means it does not help your body run at all. You are just drinking calories! It does not even become usable energy for your body to use!

Another important note to keep in mind is that alcohol does eat muscle. What does that mean exactly? If you drink alcohol, it can eat away at your muscle and make you actually lose muscle. Is that not sad? You put all that work into gaining some sort of muscle mass, do not ruin it by downing your body weight in alcohol, all right? That is just not a smart move, especially since alcohol does have calories. They do not just burn away as empty calories!

Here is a special tip: If you are going to work out in the morning or while fasted, consume a cup of coffee or caffeine. A cup of coffee before any exercise routine will increase your metabolism and cause you to burn more when you workout.

Plus, it gives you that energy boost you need to keep working hard. Is that not a great tip? My favorite drink from Starbucks is from the secret menu called "The Black Widow" (not to be confused with the competitive eater) which is just iced black tea and iced black coffee. It will give you a great kick and suppress any appetite you might have until you finish fasting. You are welcome! People who are devoted to their physical fitness or people who want to lose weight may want to include physical fitness training into their daily schedules.

One aspect of physical fitness training involves weight training, which is essential for building a faster metabolism because while the body is at rest, it will burn more if the body contains more muscle. That means you are able to eat more to maintain your body weight! Who does not want that? If you lift weights that are heavy enough to create some difficulty for you, you can build more muscle and even get your heart pumping. An elevated heart rate means you are burning more!

Here is a little advice for you, just because I care: Do not forget leg day! First of all, the muscles in your legs are amongst the largest in your body. You know that muscle you loved to say as a child? Yes, the gluteus Maximus! The gluteus Maximus is the largest muscle in the body. If you do not work it out, you are missing out on training one of the major muscles and you are severely limiting your metabolic potential!

Do not handicap yourself by forgetting such a great muscle. Second of all, have you ever seen those guys at the gym that workout their upper body almost every single day but look a little off kilter? Yeah, well, they forgot leg day. They typically have skinny looking legs that make their bodies so off balance. I have a friend who only works out the muscles he sees so typically his legs and certain parts of his upper body are smaller.

Do not be that guy. Do not forget to evenly train your muscles! Balance is key! It gets a whole lot harder to fix that once you have developed a lot in one area but are underdeveloped in another. Performing cardio is also essential to weight loss. It can create a large calorie deficit if you put the effort into it, but it is also very good for your heart. Heart health can be maintained by proper cardio. While I do not agree that you should utilize cardio for your weight loss because a number of dislike people have associated with cardio which will only lead to more distaste for cardio in the future, I do believe that cardiovascular fitness in maintaining proper health so even if your goal is not to lose weight, I think it is important to continue performing cardio, but in moderate quantities.

Do not make yourself hate cardio by forcing yourself through long episodes of cardio workouts, which I know all too well. Studies have gone back and forth on many aspects of physical fitness and weight loss, but if you want to optimize your fat loss, perform your cardio after your weight training. If you perform your weight training after your cardio workouts, you may find you have expended most of your energy so you cannot properly perform as well as you could have. Although it is important to warm up your muscles, do not tire them out with a long cardio workout.

Aside from optimizing your workouts, if you do perform your cardio workouts after your weight lifting workouts, your body has been proven to burn more fat than if you were to reverse the order of your workout, so if the idea did not entice you at first, at least you can look forward to burning more fat with this workout routine!

Think of that as a secret workout life hack! You are welcome! Of course, your body does require a certain amount of calories to properly operate. If you are at a constant caloric deficit while weight training, all you can attempt to do is keep the amount of muscle you have. You will not be gaining any muscle through a caloric deficit, so if you are trying to lose weight, you will find at the end of your weight loss period, your body will gain weight on the same amount of calories you were consuming before when you were maintaining your weight.

It is a very sad fact of dieting. An important note to take is that you should not be training extraneously when fasted. That is not to say that you cannot work out when you are fasting. Studies have gone back and forth regarding fat loss with fasted workouts. Like I said earlier, all that matters is if the calories you expend is more than the calories you intake. If your body does not perform well starved, do not work out fasted! It works for some but not all. If you do train fasted, though, you should make sure to eat a proper meal sometime after you train.

Make sure that your meal is balanced so you have protein or muscle repair and carbohydrates for energy. While I do not truly believe that your muscles can become "catabolic," it is important to eat to restore your energy. I hate when I feel completely fatigued the rest of the day after working out! I did state earlier that I do train early mornings before work, but still continue to fast after. I have not noticed a large amount of muscle loss at all unless my intake decreases drastically. I prefer to work out in the mornings because the gym is less crowded, I can just get my workout out of the way and go on with my life. Also, statistics show that if you schedule your workouts in the morning, you will most likely perform them compared to if your workouts are in the evenings, which, through experience, I can attest to.

Anyway, I fast until later in the day to prevent myself from binge eating. Training fasted also makes my cardio sessions easier since there is nothing to hinder me or make me feel lethargic. This was mainly through trial and error, but that is how my body responds. Like I have expressed often throughout this book, you should do what works best for your body! All of our bodies do not function or react the same! With that in mind, you must tailor your workouts according to how your body reacts. Some people develop certain body parts a lot faster. For me, my calves develop fairly quickly, which I can tell by the immense pain in my shins when I run. Some people's glutes may grow faster, but some people may not grow muscle easily at all.

This does not just apply to muscles. Some bodies just burn fat faster and not gain any easily, while others gain fat quickly and cannot even get the fat off. It just is not fair, is it? You just need to figure out what type of body you have and figure out what types of workouts work best for you. We may not be all gifted genetically, but that does not mean we cannot do anything about it!

Chapter 7: Intermittent Fasting Types

Intermittent fasting can take several forms. The person designing the method usually determines the difference. However, the factor of fasting and eating will be the constant. All methods have their rewards, so it doesn't really matter, which method you adopt. Therefore, go for the one that you feel more comfortable with and that you feel you can achieve.

The probability of you adhering to the rules is higher if you pick one that you are comfortable with. For beginners, it is advised that you go for a shorter fasting window and a longer eating window. Your body might take between two to four weeks to fully adapt to the new eating system and this is the point where you have to be strong to resist temptations and avoid all those cravings.

Most individuals are already used to eating whenever it suits them so engaging in IF can be really stressful especially at the starting period. Your appetite will naturally lessen once your body adapts to the new eating system. You will also feel a lot slimmer, energetic and alert as you go further. Here are some of the IF techniques:

Fasting Method Number 1

Martin Berkhan designed the first one. His method is quite easy to maintain and very popular. The rule of his technique is that women and men will have 10 and 8 hours eating window respectively, thus leaving them with 14 and 16 hours fasting window. Positive results can be hindered by inconsistent feeding windows thus it is vital to maintaining the windows.

Martin is of the opinion that meals should be consumed around the workout periods. For instance, if 7 pm is supposed to be the end of your feeding window, 5:30 pm should be a good time for workout and meals. Or you could end your fasting windows with workouts that way, you will be able to consume the nutrients required to replenish lost ones just after your workout.

Fasting Method Number 2

The next technique is the Ori Hofmekeler's Warrior Diet. This method could be considered more difficult. In this technique, you are only allowed to eat once a day, which is at night. You are expected to fast for 20 hours per day. Presumably, our ancestors survived doing this.

Although it is impossible to know for sure whether our ancestors did this or not, this method remains very effective. Major positive differences have been recorded by individuals who have engaged themselves in this method. This method might not be the best to start off with; however, the Marin's method would be better for beginners and after a while, you can reduce your eating window till you have just 4 hours left.

You must understand that this method does not allow for small in between meals and as such, don't dive into the deep end of the pool only to struggle to keep up with the 4 hours of eating window. There are certain guiding rules on what you can and cannot eat. This is one of the stricter methods of Intermittent Fasting and as such, you will have to maintain the approved food options, this method is very difficult and as such it is not recommended as much as the others.

Fasting Method Number 3

The third is the method designed by Brad Pilo and is known as the Eat Stop Eat method. This program is a bestseller on the internet. This method basically asks that a complete 24 hour fast be done 2 or 3 times in one week. During the period when you are not fasting, you are allowed to eat whatever you wish. Doing this, you will consume fewer calories and lose weight as a result of this. You can still eat your favorite foods; however, it should be on a day that you are not fasting.

For those who do not want to let go of their favorite meals, this is a huge relief. Notwithstanding, it can be really difficult to go for 24 hours without food. Just as stated earlier, Martin's method is very good for beginners from where you can work your way up.

How do you decide among these methods?

The fact that a method works for someone around you doesn't mean it will work for you. Tailor your fast to suit yourself and while doing this, you must take into consideration your job requirements, sleeping patterns, eating habits etc.

It is always better to allow your sleeping hours fall within your fasting window and you can wait up to six hours after waking up to start your eating window. That is if you are into Martin's method. Some other social commitments can make IF really difficult to maintain.

Whether you like it or not, your social life will be affected by your fasting. Here, you need to be smart to make it work for you. Take for example, Hugh Jackman was on IF while practicing for the movie – Wolverine. Despite the rigors of such schedule, he stuck to his IF program.

It often feels like torture and some people give up and just grab something to eat. This can lead to a feeling of guilt or it may leave you feeling like you failed. They have failed because their goals were not realistic. Setting reasonable goals and marking measurable success is vital to achieving success.

Chapter 8: Intermittent Fasting Plan

The fact that various people have different needs makes it extremely difficult to give you an IF plan. However, you can use the following guides to plan your program.

Know Your Goals.

You should be aware of your calorie number and how many calories you are to consume in order to maintain the caloric deficit of about 500 per day, that is if you want to adopt the IF plan. You are to maintain a caloric surplus if you wish to build your body; however, all calories needed must be consumed during the eating window. It is harder to consume lots of calories because of the time frame by which you have to consume the food but if you are able to consume a lot of calories it is not likely that you will gain fat, if you are in the intermittent fasting program.

You can continue eating what you are eating at the moment if you are okay with your weight level, just ensure your meals are consumed during the eating window. In other words if you want to maintain your current weight but get healthier, keep the same calorie intake that you currently have but adopt the intermittent schedule. If you want to lose weight adopt the intermittent fasting program and reduce your current calorie input by 500 calories. And if you want to gain muscle, make sure that while exercising you maintain the intermittent fasting program and increase your calorie intake by 500 calories a day.

Know Your Schedule.

 Timing is the major focus of intermittent fasting and not particularly what you eat. For you to effectively do the IF plan, your eating period and cut-off time must be strictly adhered to. The eating and fasting windows usually control the lives of those involved in IF. They constantly have to check their time and plan accordingly.

Proper planning can help to avoid all these inconveniences. Consider your preferences and schedule: When do you get out of bed? When is the lunch break at your office? Would you rather fast before night sleep or after the morning after the night sleep? You can design your eating window to start 6 hours after you wake up if you would rather go to bed with a full stomach. What happens when you get hungry at work? Will you have the opportunity to take a break and have a meal when the eating window begins? You must consider all these before setting your IF plan.

How Many Meals Will You Eat?

Whatever you like, factor it into your plan. Some would rather have one or two big meals during their eating window while some others may prefer to eat little meals all through the eating window. When Are You Working Out?

A regular exercise program is advised. However, you must factor this into your plan. Do you want to train on a full stomach or on an empty one? It is usually better to have your meal after workouts because this way, the body can regain lost energy and the fuel needed for metabolism can be obtained from the meals.

Chapter 9: Methods of Intermittent Fasting

It is generally accepted that there are 5 methods that can be used for effective fasting. These have either been put together by diet gurus or by scientists and are thought to be effective for their own reasons. As everybody is different it may be that you find one method more appealing than another or that one method will work better for you. Since individually it is hard to tell which this is it will be something you may have to try for yourself before getting results.

Method 1: Leangains

This method is intended for those who spend a lot of time in the gym, it focuses on losing fat and building muscle and was created by Martain Berkhan. If you aren't trying to gain muscle this might be a problem because many who want to lose weight do not want to become muscular.

The program advocates fasting for 14-16 hours a day though during this time you are allowed black coffee, sugar-free gum, calorie free soda and water. Essentially you are allowing yourself very tiny amounts of calories the FDA considers any product that has less than 5 calories a serving as being calorie free since your body needs to consume more than that to process the food. Most people find the easiest way to follow this is simply too fast through the night and morning, though they are still able to have their morning coffee as usual.

During the remaining 6-8 hours participants can "feed" and this will change depending on what days you exercise. On the days where you work out you will need to consume a higher level of carbs while on rest days you will need a higher level of fats. Your protein consumption should remain constant and high – the expected level is approximately 20g/day. If you aren't a nutritionist it is easy to see where an app like Calorie Counter might be essential until you get the hang of things. The foods you consume should also be whole and unprocessed as much as possible though this is a basic understanding of any healthy diet.

There are some pros and cons to this method. Firstly if you don't have time for a meal the program allows you to have a protein or nutritional shake instead though this is not intended to be a regular feature since it can push your body too far by having too few calories.

Another benefit is that there is no set meal time within the feeding schedule you may eat the entire 6-8 hour span within reason though many will still schedule 2-3 meals within that time.

Though so far you might think this is an easy program the emphasis with lean gains is what you eat. The guidelines within what you can eat are fairly strict and you will need to go over them in depth to make sure all your foods are within that parameter.

Time Windows

It is up to you to choose when your time window takes place, but it is recommended to time it smart and stay consistent with your time window. It is important to keep it sustainable, so you need to set the time window on moments that suit you well. For example, if you are someone who goes to the gym every morning, it will not be very smart to stuff yourself full right before you go.

Or if you are someone who has a 9-5 job, I wouldn't recommend taking in all your calories while you are working, as this can prevent you from staying focused on your work. Also, we are creatures of habit, so use this to your advantage.

Decide beforehand on which moment your time window will start each day, and stay consistent with that time window! Sticking to the program will be harder when you aren't consistent, due to the fact that you are repeatedly breaking the habit and because you aren't giving yourself the opportunity to form the habit in the first place.

Types of Food

What type of foods you eat depends on your goals, body fat, age and gender. Generally, you should eat a lot of protein, even on non-workout days. However, don't consume too much, as this could lead to protein toxicity. It is important to eat more carbohydrates than fats on training days, but lower your overall carbohydrate consumption when you are trying to lose body fat. Regardless of your goals, you should eat whole and unprocessed foods the majority of the time. You can occasionally have cheat days, but do this in moderation.

Benefits of Leangains

• Saves Money

When you are skipping certain meals for breakfast and lunch, this will provide a good opportunity to save money. Many people underestimate the amount of money they spend on breakfast and lunch every day.

• No Counting Calories

When you choose to eat in a short time window or eat all of your calories in one or two meals, it will become extremely hard to consume too many calories (if you are not eating junk food). Therefore, you will save yourself the trouble of micromanaging your calorie intake every time.

• Burns Fat

When you are following the Leangains diet, you will automatically eat less carbohydrates than normal. This will result in burning a lot of body fat. Your body will adapt to the fact that you aren't eating a lot of carbohydrates and it will burn the fat you have in order to receive energy.

Cons of Leangains

Leangains provides much flexibility when it comes to when you eat, but is very strict in the kind of foods you can eat. Most of the time this won't be a problem for active gym addicts, because the most committed are disciplined when it comes to nutrition.

Method 2: The Warrior Diet

This diet is ideal for those who like to outperform and dedicate to their goals. The language of the diet is very simple and the process even simpler. This is great for those who are very busy or who don't want to expend any time or effort adjusting their life to a diet. This diet has no feeding periods, or restrictions and is geared more towards those who feel comfortable undereating. In fact the problem with the Warrior Diet is that many people may find themselves in starvation as it is too extreme for those who aren't in the average range.

The program involves a 20 day fast and then a 4 hour period in which to eat a single large meal. However, during the 20 days fast you are allowed a few servings of raw veggies, fresh juice, and lean protein if desired. In this way this isn't a traditional fasting diet like the others because you aren't wholly fasting and can consume food during the fast period. The intention here is that the undereating promotes alertness by affecting the Sympathetic Nervous System.

The overeating period that follows this maximizes the recuperation from the fast without causing the body to go into starvation since you have consumed minimal calories to keep the metabolism going. The program advocates eating at night to make the body produce hormones and burn fat during the day as much as possible. According to Ori Hofmekler, who created the diet, the order in which you eat foods during your food groups is more important than anything during the four hour period. He advocates eating vegetables, followed by proteins, and then fats and only then if you are hungry resorting to carbohydrates.

This is by far one of the most popular fasting diets as it still allows participants to eat during the fasting period and isn't a true fast. Many have also said they really do feel more alert and have more energy by practicing this method. It seems this diet has a lot more pros than the others but yet again it falls short in that the eating period is quite strict, especially the order of eating. In addition it is also easy to overeat or at the very least consume far too many calories since you are eating during the day and then eating a bigger meal at night.

If your BMR is quite low this might be a disaster for you since you could eat enough calories grazing during the day that your "large" evening meal isn't necessary. The strict scheduling can also cause problems socially since you may not be able to eat with others or have to eat in a different order. It's also going to be difficult to follow if you don't like large meals or don't like to eat a lot at night.

Benefits of the Warrior Diet

• Eating Snacks in the Fasting Windows

One of the main benefits of this diet is that you can occasionally eat in your fasting window. You can consume fruits, veggies and fruit juice.

• Very Healthy

Another benefit of this diet is that you are getting all the nutrients you need on a daily basis. Cons of the Warrior Diet This diet can be very hard to sustain due to the fact that it is very strict on when and what to eat. Not many people can afford to eat at night, and some people find it very hard to consistently eat healthily.

Method 3: Eat and Stop

This method is quite difficult for those beginning fasting, especially if one of the reasons you have for being overweight is grazing. The stop phase of this program involves a 24 hour fast, and though at the beginning you are allowed to acclimatize to it eventually you are expected to go for the full 24 hours.

The idea behind this is that you are restricting your overall weekly calorie intake without having to limit what you're eating at all the rest of the time. This program also advocates resistance training as an exercise to maximize benefits. Similarly to the Leangains program you are still allowed calorie-free drinks like diet soda and coffee though no gum. There is no set schedule here so you can time your fast however you please – if you choose to finish your fast with a meal or a small snack is unimportant as long as you have completed the 24 hour period.

Though 24 hours may seem excessive the flexibility of this program can make this an easier program for beginners since you have no food restrictions. The creator, Brad Pilon, suggests spending the first day fasting for as long as you can before eating and then gradually extending that time each week until you reach your goal. He also suggests starting the fast at a time when you are busy so that you don't notice your lack of eating so much. Though there is no set dietary requirements it is still expected that you will eat healthy on your non-fasting days and the 24 hours is simply intended as and extra boost to lowering your calories on the other days.

The biggest con of this method is obviously the extended time without food. Most people will struggle with headaches, stomach cramps, fatigue, and becoming obnoxious simply because of hunger. In fact many people do get angry and cranky when hungry so it can be tempting to binge to get rid of this but this period is all about self-control. If you are nervous about how well you can control yourself over this period then this diet may be too challenging to follow. In other words this isn't meant for the casual dieter, this is more aimed towards those who already have a healthy lifestyle but need an extra boost to get to their weight loss goals.

Benefits of Eat Stop Eat

• Calorie Deficit Without Willpower Usage

Because you are limiting eating for just one or two days, it won't require any (or a lot of) willpower. When you know that you can eat what you want after enduring the 24-hour fast, it will be much easier to stick to it.

• Eat What You Want

You can also eat what you want, when you want, so this will help to prevent those nasty binges. The only thing is, moderation is key. You should only consume bad foods in moderation. Having one or two hands of chips is totally fine, but eating a bag of chips a day is not.

Cons of Eat Stop Eat

It can be hard to be disciplined in the Eat Stop Eat diet, even when you can eat what you want. Some people have a hard time eating bad food in moderation or binge on the days they can eat. If you find yourself struggling with a lack of self-control, then I wouldn't recommend this method to you.

Method 4: Up Day Down/The Alternate Day Diet

This is probably the easiest plan of the five here and is designed for those aiming to reach and maintain a specific goal. The program advocates eating very little one day followed by a normal intake the next day. If you are using the average 2000 calorie day as a guide this would mean your fast day should be between 400 to 500 calories. There is also a conveniently available tool online from the Dr. James Johnson who created the diet to calculate this based on your needs.

The doctor also advocates meal replacement products like shakes and bars on low-calorie days to maximize your nutritional intake on those. These products are also easier to ration out during the day than trying to calculate food amounts and needs then breaking them down to ration. The idea behind this is that once you have started to get the hang of rationing yourself, you can begin to transition over to regular foods on your fast days while still keeping in the guided amount.

As a method this is the most well supported,probably because it has been formulated by a doctor. This program gives you the necessary ~30% calorie reduction while giving you about a 1-2% weight loss per week (around 2lb for most people). However it can be easy to "forget" you're dieting on those alternate days which could cause binging and the diet to fail. The plan does advocate meal planning as well so that you don't find yourself in this situation or being forced into fast food.

One of the most notable differences with this diet is that it does not advocate fast results but a more sustained rate over time, this can be frustrating and many will feel they are not getting results or that the diet isn't working.

Each of these methods has pros and cons, and with any weight loss method you may not see immediate results which is why it is important to stick with it. If you struggle with the timing of the meals or cannot stretch yourself to fast for as long as the diets require you can also consider programs like the Primal Diet or Intuitive eating. Eat WHEN for example trains dieters to listen to when their body gives them cues about when to eat. If you're a grazer by nature though this is an easy path to overeating and it may simply be time to master your willpower and work with an intermittent fasting method.

Benefits of this method

• Rapid Weight Loss

Due the fact that you are cutting a lot of calories every day, you will see results very fast. Many people report that they lose about 1-2 pounds a week.

• Eat What You Prefer

There is no restriction on what to eat, but it is advised to eat unprocessed and whole foods. However, you may only eat the maximum amount of calories you need to maintain your weight on the normal calorie days.

• Doesn't Require Much Willpower

Because you are only cutting calories for 2-3 days a week, you won't use too much willpower. It can be difficult at first, but it is better to start the diet very small. Start by cutting a few calories out on the low-calorie days and gradually keep increasing this.

Method 5: Fast/Feast method

If you're a fan of cheat days this could be the one for you, the other diets have advocated snacking or drinks as cheats during your fasting period while this one actually combines all three and then still allows you one cheat day a week. The rest of the week is then split up using different methods of fasting. As with the EatStopEat program the creators suggest using your busiest time as your fasting period so you don't realize you're fasting as much.

Unlike the other plans, however this one also has a companion training program for participants to maximize the results they have as easily as possible. In this way even though you aren't following as strict of a dietary regime it is a higher impact on your lifestyle since you will need to follow an exercise regime too. The biggest bonus of using this method is that for those who aren't good at planning out or scheduling eating times this program has everything already scheduled out for you. Conveniently this allows you to have your cheat day while still giving you structure and maximum rewards.

The opposite of this is that one cheat day can often turn into two and then the whole program fails so though it doesn't require as much willpower as EatStopEat it does mean that you will need enough to keep your cheating in check. Also since the planned schedule varies on a daily basis there is not a lot of room for flexibility and it can be inconvenient to fit into a busy lifestyle. The calendar provided with the program will provide some help but it is still the largest impact on your day compared to the other programs.

Benefits of this method

• Fat Loss

By fasting for 36 hours, you are taking in a lower amount of calories. This will lead to a rapid fat loss.

• Full Cheat Days

The Fast/Feast Model allows you to implement full cheat days. This is excellent for the common sweet tooth and it helps you to keep your metabolism working.

• Removes Food Cravings

By implementing cheat days, it becomes easier to resist unhealthy foods along the way. It will give your body a mental and physical break. Removing food cravings will help you to avoid overeating junk food.

Cons of Eat Stop Eat

The method is relatively difficult to follow due to the following two reasons:

1) Very Difficult To Keep Your Calories In Check

For most people it will become very difficult to keep their calories in check during their cheat days. If you are unfamiliar with the amount of calories that most foods contain, it is almost impossible to not cross your limit too much.

2) 36-Hour Fasts Can Be Very Long

If you have never fasted before, it can be very difficult to sustain the 36-hour fast. Most people who do this version of Intermittent Fasting are already familiar and advanced with it, which is why they are able to sustain it easier.

However, like the Alternate Day Diet, start this model by beginning small. Don't try to fast for 36 hours at once, but rather begin small by fasting for 12 hours and gradually increase the time.

Chapter 10: Efficiency in Intermittent Fasting

I remember that when I started, I made some critical mistakes which slowed down the process of implementing Intermittent Fasting. I want to show you exactly how to implement Intermittent Fasting efficiently without making unnecessary mistakes.

Step #1: Start With The Why

With everything you do in life, you should know the reasons behind it. Doing certain things without knowing exactly why you are doing them will eventually cause you to fail. The same goes with Intermittent Fasting. Before you even start to implement it, you need to know why you want to implement Intermittent Fasting. Our Different Personalities Ok, how do you do this? We human beings have different personalities (or different selves). We have a lower, a standard and a higher self. We tend to switch between these personalities throughout the day, depending on the time, place, situation and environment we are in.

Every one of these personalities is motivated by different things and you need to align all these personalities to the same goal: implementing Intermittent Fasting. And when your goal (to implement Intermittent Fasting) is not aligned between these personalities, you will eventually sabotage yourself. Therefore, the key is to come up with reasons that are emotionally compelling to you for all your personalities to achieve a particular goal.

For example, let's say that you are in a standard mood; you suddenly decide to lose 10 pounds of body fat and your motivation is because you want to look good. You realize that you need to change your eating patterns, so you go on a diet. Well, it is very good to go on a diet, and "looking good" is a very good reason to lose body fat. However, there is one problem… you only know why your standard self-wants to lose 10 pounds of body fat. But what about your higher self or your lower self? Why do 'they' want to lose the body fat? What if you catch yourself in a stressed-out mood and crave some junk food? You will most likely think "screw this diet" and sabotage yourself. Or when you are in a higher self, you don't specifically care about looking good, so you think "why to bother?"

How To Recognize Our Different Personalities

So again, the key is to come up with reasons that are emotionally compelling to you for all your personalities. And how do you recognize your different selves? Simple, by the thought patterns you have. Normally, when you have negative thought patterns, you tend to be in your lower self. When you have neutral thoughts, you are in your standard self, and if you have very positive thoughts, you are in your higher self. Your Lower Self: Tends to be motivated by selfish, irrational and slightly more childish reasons being better than others, showing people a lesson, being lazy, avoiding responsibility etc.

Your Standard Self: Tends to be motivated by logical, rational and ethical reasons like: knowing that you need to do XYZ to get a certain result, realizing your responsibility etc.

Your Higher Self: Tends to be motivated by a sense of higher purpose like: motivating and inspiring others, having a positive impact on the world, contributing to society etc.

Exercise: Determine Your Own Reasons To Implement Intermittent Fasting

Now that you know how to create your own reasons for implementing Intermittent Fasting, it is time for you to determine them. Take 10 minutes to a half hour to sit down and come up with all the reasons why you want/ need to implement Intermittent Fasting. I have showed you all the benefits of Intermittent Fasting and I also showed you that the most common myths about Intermittent Fasting simply aren't true. Now, take the time to look at the reasons which compel you the most.

Also, come up with other personal reasons to implement Intermittent Fasting. These reasons need to be emotionally compelling to you and move you towards your goal. Also, only having negative or positive reasons for implementing Intermittent Fasting is not good enough. You need to have both (and even logical reasons).

Again, take 10 minutes to a half hour to come up with reasons for your lower self, standard self and higher self. Be sure to come up with as many reasons as possible!

Step #2: Choose Which Intermittent Fasting Model You

Want To Implement, we have discussed several Intermittent Fasting Models that you can implement. These models are very similar, but differ in the actual execution. Again, which model you should implement is completely up to you, but it depends on your goals. You need to clearly define your goals and check which Intermittent Fasting model is the best choice for your personal goal.

You can, of course, also mix the concepts of these Intermittent Fasting models. For example, I have implemented a variation of the Leangains model and the Alternate Day Diet model. I really like the concept of the Leangains model, but there are some things that aren't practical for me. So, I decided to create little modifications to the model by mixing it with the Alternate Day Diet model. To be honest though, I don't recommend you create a variation of the models if you are new to Intermittent Fasting.

I recommend that you first choose a model, execute it and see what happens. If you find that it isn't practical for you, then it may be smart to make some small tweaks to the model or try to implement another one.

Step #3: Divide The Principles Of Your Chosen Model Into Habits You Can Implement

These habits are discussed in the next chapter, Chapter 11. Again, everything we human beings do in life is a learned habit. Habits can be our greatest asset or our greatest liability. For example, someone who is exercising daily has formed a great habit (read: asset). But someone who is eating junk food every day has formed a very disturbing habit (read: liability). You want to form great habits that will help you to move forward towards your goals.

But implementing these habits can be very difficult, because it demands willpower to create a habit. So what you'll want to do is to divide all the principles into tiny habits that you can implement easily. At first it will feel as if you aren't making any progress, but I can assure you that you will if you do it consistently.

Also, don't make the mistake of trying to implement too many habits at once. You have a limited amount of willpower and when you implement too many habits, you will burn through all your willpower very fast, resulting in you sabotaging your progress or discarding the whole Intermittent Fasting model.

Step #4: Review And Visualize Your Habits plus Implement One A Month

To properly implement the habits chosen in step 3, you need to implement them very slowly. I know a lot of people want to make change very quick, so they decide to overhaul their diet within a week. This is not the correct way to do it! No matter how much willpower you have, every human being has a breaking point. The breaking point is the point where you burn out all your willpower and discard all your chosen habits. When that happens, you are not making progress, or worse, you are actually going backward!

Chapter 11: Habits that can be adapted for Successful fasting

To make it easier to you, I have divided all the Intermittent Fasting models from chapter 3 into tiny habits here below:

Leangains

Habit 1: Starting your eating window on X hour (the moment you want to start your eating window daily).

Habit 2: Break your eating window on X+8 hours (8 hours after you have started your eating window).

Habit 3A (For people trying to lose weight): Eat 25% carbohydrates, 40% protein, and 35% fat of your total daily calorie consumption.

Habit 3B (For people trying to gain weight): Eat 50% carbohydrates, 35% protein, and 15% fat of your total daily calorie consumption. Make sure you eat approximately 200-400 more calories than shown to properly gain weight.

The Warrior Diet

Habit 1: Starting your eating window on X hour (the moment you want to start your eating window daily, but it has to be in the night).

Habit 2: Break your eating window on X+4 hours (4 hours after you have started your eating window).

Habit 3: Replace bad snacks (processed foods etc.) with fruits

Habit 4: Start eating small portions of the protein outside your eating window (around 100 calories per meal).

Habit 5: Replace bad drinks (soft drinks etc.) with fruit juice and water.

Eat Stop Eat

Habit 1: Choose a day where you want to fast for 24 hours and start by fasting for 12 hours on that day.

Habit 2: Increase your fast to 16 hours on that day.

Habit 3: Increase your fast to 20 hours on that day.

Habit 4: Increase your fast to 24 hours on that day.

Habit 5 (for people who want to fast for 24 hours on another day): Repeat habit #1 to habit #4 for another day.

Alternate Day Diet

First, determine how many calories you need to sustain your weight.

Habit 1: Make sure that you consume the amount of calories needed to sustain your weight every day.

Habit 2: Eat 80% of your calories on low-calorie days.

Habit 3: Decrease that to 60% of your calories on low-calorie days.

Habit 4: Decrease that to 40% of your calories on low-calorie days.

Habit 5: Decrease that to 20% of your calories on low-calorie days.

Fast/Feast Model

Habit 1: Endure a 12-hour fast followed by a normal day of eating

Habit 2: Endure an 18-hour fast followed by a normal day of eating

Habit 3: Endure a 24-hour fast followed by a normal day of eating

Habit 4: Endure a 32-hour fast followed by a cheat day

Habit 5: Endure a 36-hour fast followed by a cheat day
How to Implement A Habit

So how do you implement habits without burning out all your willpower?

Implement one habit a month. For example, decide that you are going to execute habit 1 on day 1 all the way to day 30. If you have done that successfully, you may proceed to implement habit 2. If you catch yourself failing to execute habit 1 somewhere between day 1 and day 30, restart the cycle. I know that it sounds very boring and annoying to do, but this is the only way to do it effectively.

Also, realize that the more you do something, the easier it gets. Only the first week or two will be the toughest, and after that you can be almost 100% sure that you will follow through.

Another thing to consider is that if you have implemented the first habit successfully, but you catch yourself failing to execute it while trying to implement habit 2, you need to go back and start the 30 days over with habit 1.

The goal is not to do every habit for 30 days once, but rather to sustain those habits. Therefore, always make sure that the habits you implemented earlier are being carried out while doing the newer ones.

Review and Visualize Your Habits.

Also, you need to take approximately 10 minutes a day to effectively review and visualize yourself doing the habits. If you do this, you will constantly remind yourself why you are doing what you are doing and help yourself to make the habit a part of your reality.

To effectively review your habit, read the reasons why you want to implement those habits. After that, take 7-10 minutes to visualize doing the habit successfully.

Chapter 12: What can cause failure in Intermittent Fasting

Many people may fail to sustain fasting. In this chapter, we are going to look at some of the factors that may cause individuals to be unsuccessful in making a good and required fast.

Reason #1: Your Reasons Aren't Strong Enough

As stated earlier, you need to come up with several compelling reasons to implement Intermittent Fasting into your life. If you don't have enough reasons that emotionally compel you at all times, you will be more likely to fail. Also, there is a chance that people will question your decision and if you aren't able to fully explain to yourself exactly why you need to implement Intermittent Fasting, at some point you will think: "Why bother? Screw this."

Solution:

The solution is very simple - state at least 15 reasons that emotionally compel you on why you should Intermittent Fast. This will help you to stick to it, even when people question your behavior.

Reason #2: Going Too Hard

Even if you are doing everything right, the chances are that you are still failing to sustain your Intermittent Fasting diet. Why? Because you are trying to implement all the habits at once. While I understand that you want to implement Intermittent Fasting into your life quickly, it isn't the smartest way to go about it. We as human beings have a limited amount of willpower, and every time you try to implement a new habit, you use up a bit.

So, you can understand that if you try to implement them all at once, you will deplete all of your willpower very quickly. When this happens, you have reached your breaking point. When you have reached your breaking point, you will most likely give up on Intermittent Fasting and go back in doing things the old way. Or worse, you there will be a chance that you will develop bad habits.

Solution:

As discussed earlier, you need to identify whether you are a slow learner or a fast learner. How fast are you able to implement things? This is a question you can only answer by experimenting with it. Begin small and gradually, then increase a number of habits you take on.

Realize that everyone has a breaking point and everyone will give up when they have reached this breaking point. If you catch yourself giving up eventually, even while doing everything right, choose to apply the habits a bit slower than you had planned to. See the implementation of Intermittent Fasting as a marathon, not a sprint.

Slow but steady will always win the race. It is the person who implements things slowly but consistently who succeeds, as opposed to the person who goes all out for the first 2 weeks and quits after that. In short, take it one step at a time and stay consistent.

Reason #3 Too Many Distractions

To quote Jim Rohn, "You are the average of the 5 people you spend the most time with." With this quote, Jim Rohn is trying to say that you will take on the habits of the people you spend the most time with, whether you like it or not. This is because we human beings are social creatures and one of our primal desires is to belong to a group of people.

But also (as discussed earlier), you just have as much willpower that you can use to sustain your own habits when you are with these 5 people. If you are someone who eats healthy all the time, but your 5 people are junk food addicts, it won't take too long until you catch yourself eating junk food regularly.

These 5 people can be a blessing or a curse to your goals. If they have the same goals as you, it will become a lot easier to succeed. If this is not the case, you will set yourself up for failure. Therefore, there might be a chance that you aren't able to stick with Intermittent Fasting due to these people.

Solution:

The first thing you need to realize is that it isn't their fault that you aren't succeeding with Intermittent Fasting. It is just that your and their goals are in conflict. A way to get around this is by asking them if they want to help you with the issue. Explain to them why Intermittent Fasting is so important to you and show them what results it brings you. Ask them if they can respect your decision and whether they can eat at different moments if you are around.

I personally asked my friends to bear in mind that it was very difficult for me to stick to fasting when they would consistently eat around me, and I rarely had any issues with them. Even the individual who stated that it was a waste of my time was still able to respect me by eating elsewhere when I was around. If some people really don't want to cooperate, choose to remove yourself from their presence when they eat. In short, eliminate all distractions. As stated earlier, you need to come up with several compelling reasons to implement Intermittent Fasting into your life. If you don't have enough reasons that emotionally compel you at all times, you will be more likely to fail.

Conclusion

Congratulations, you've reached the end of Intermittent Fasting! I hope you know a lot more about fasting and that you (if you haven't already) will start implementing Intermittent Fasting into your life. Now that you know that fasting provides a lot of benefits, is easy to implement and that the common myths aren't true, I hope you are motivated to implement the information.

The truth is with intermittent fasting there really isn't one as it is much easier to do than it first seems. To lose weight with intermittent fasting you don't change your healthy eating habits at all except for one or two 24 hour periods each week where you don't consume any calories. These facts should be scheduled to make them as easy as possible. When not fasting you just eat what you normally would. Ideally this should feature good quality meats and fish with mostly fibrous, not starchy or sweet carbohydrates plus a lot of drinking water. Just don't eat waste your fast be eating extra to make up for it! Don't fast more than twice per week or for longer than 24 hours at any one time.

The intermittent fasting program can be very effective, safe and sustainable. One of the best benefits of IF is that once you have the program in place you can carry it on for life. You do not need special food or to buy special supplements or a special program, you can eat what you normally eat just at a scheduled timeframe.

Unlike a fad diet, which only works for a short period of time, the intermittent fasting method can be a lifestyle. You can eat real food and get all the nutrients you need. There are no restrictions. A key to remember with any program is that there are no true shortcuts, all the programs at the beginning will be difficult because they are forcing you to change. But with the intermittent fasting method if you stick to it and make it your lifestyle you will not have the problem of the yo-yo effect (going up and down in weight).

One thing that I recommend is that you should always consult with a physician or nutritionist before starting this or any program that involves changes in your nutrition or involves a change in your exercise regimen.

Thank you for taking the time to join me in this in this journey of understanding intermittent fasting. Fasting can make people achieve a lot in life. So know the essence of taking a fast and good luck in all your fasting endeavors.

Thank you again for downloading this book!